I0425482

Copyright © 2019

Table of Contents

Introduction

When we hear the word, 'keto', our minds usually dwell on weight loss. Keto is far more than that. The creators of the diet had the mind of using it to treat epilepsy, and it worked effortlessly well. Once better anticonvulsant medications came on board, its usage reduced. Over the years, it was noticed that keto could do more than treat epilepsy, it can help in the treatment of Alzheimer's disease and even shed weight.

A lot of persons have embraced the diet as one that allows them to remain fit, and lose weight without stress, though some sacrifices have to be made. You have to wat healthily. One thing that makes the keto diet stand out from the rest is that you don't have to sacrifice your need for sweet things and eat only bland foods.

You will have to toss those sweets that are high in carbs and sugar, but you can embrace keto sweets and snacks that are delicious and sugar-free. Who said your craving couldn't be cured in a ketogenic lifestyle?

Chapter One

Understanding what the Ketogenic diet is

The ketogenic diet is a diet that has a high amount of fats, moderate amount of protein and low amounts of carbs. All three features have to be there. Eating low carbs foods while eating foods high in protein can't be described as keto. This is because eating foods that are high in protein are similar to eating high carbs foods. When the body has excess protein, it turns it to glucose. The fats have to be high; the protein has to be moderate, while the carbs have to be low.

Ketogenic diet started when researchers in the early 1920s wanted to mimic the same effects that fasting had on epilepsy. It was noticed then that when a person fasted, the seizure he had reduced. Scientists wanted to do the same thing without people going without foods. It was noticed that the effects were replicated. Those kids that had epilepsy noticed that their seizures reduced, even after they stopped taking the diet. When good anticonvulsant medications came out, the need for a keto diet to treat epilepsy reduced.

In the case of weight loss, it is noticed that fasting can get us to the state of ketosis. This is the main reason we do a ketogenic diet. We want to be in the state of ketosis. At this state, the body turns the stored up fats to ketones, and use it as an energy source. When someone fasts, the person tends to use up stored up fats, but it is unhealthy. It is advisable to avoid fasting and opt for a safer means of getting into the state of ketosis, through a ketogenic diet.

Your body is given the nutrients it needs to survive while you lose weight. This is a classic case of killing two birds with a stone.

Chapter Two

Are You On A Ketogenic Diet?

It is common to hear a lot of persons complain that they don't know if they are in the state of ketosis. While on the journey to losing weight through a ketogenic diet, one thing is sure you can easily tell if you have reached the state of ketosis. Bellows are ways to tell:

1. Increased ketones

If you want to be sure if you are in a state of ketosis, you can draw a blood sample and take it for a test. The blood sample will tell how high your ketone levels are.

When you have a high amount of ketones in your body, you are in a state of ketosis. A breathalyzer can also pick up from your breath if you are in a state of ketosis. You can get the doctor to run a test on your urine to see your level of ketosis. Urine and breath tests aren't as reliable as the blood test.

If you don't want to test it in the hospital, you can get a home testing kit that can show you the levels of blood ketones. If you are in the nutritional ketosis, you should have ketones of about 0.5–3 millimoles per liter.

You can opt for indicator strips to see the levels of the urine. Buy your ketone testing kits online, and run the test at home.

2. Weight loss

This is one symptom that you will notice. You don't need any test kit to tell you that you have lost weight. When you are in ketosis, you should notice your body shedding weight.

This is because your body no longer has access to a high amount of carbs. Hence it has to use the stored up fats as energy. It first turns the stored up fats to ketones.

If you are in a state of ketosis, you should be losing weight.

3. Thirst

When you are in a state of ketosis, you start to notice that you are very thirsty. This is usually because you are losing water. When you are in a state of ketosis, you urinate a lot and need water. Hence you are a lot thirsty.

When you have a high amount of ketones in your body, you will notice that you are shedding a lot of water and electrolytes.

It is advisable that you drink a lot of water and liquids while on a keto diet. You need to balance the water that you are constantly losing.

4. Muscle cramps and spasms

When you are dehydrated a lot of suffering from the electrolyte imbalances, you will notice that your muscles are suffering from cramps. The electrolytes that you lose during keto are those things that transport the electrical signals from one cell to the other.

When these substances are low, you will notice that the electrical messages aren't passing well, and this could lead to spasms and muscle contractions.

It is advisable to drink a lot of water and liquids to avoid the symptoms of imbalance.

5. Headaches

When you are in a state of ketosis, you will notice that you have headaches. This isn't the case of every one. Why does this happen? Usually, this headache lasts for a day but less than a week.

The headaches are caused because your body is trying to adapt to the keto diet. Since you are consuming little carbs, the body has to adapt to the new energy source, ketones.

It could also be caused by electrolyte imbalances and dehydration. Whatever you do, consume a lot of water and liquids.

If you notice that your headache passes three days, see your doctor immediately, as it happens only at the initial stage of keto.

6. Fatigue and weakness

When a person is starting a ketogenic diet, there is a tendency of the person feeling weak. This occurs because the body is adapting to burning ketones instead of glucose. Glucose usually gives a quick burst of energy, unlike ketones. In a few days, the tiredness disappears because your body adapts to ketones. After a while on the keto diet, your energy level will increase, and you may need even more energy than someone that's not on the keto diet.

If you don't notice your energy coming back in a few weeks, you should consider talking to your physician.

7. Stomach complaints

When you make changes to your diet, your body starts to act up. That's the basic truth. This is why you start having stomach upsets when you travel out to a strange land and dine on exotic cuisines. You will realize that you have tummy complaints. Your body is not yet used to the food, but after a while, the stomach complaints stop because your body has adjusted. The same can be said for the ketogenic lifestyle.

You may notice some stomach complaints, but it is for a short while.

To help solve this, you should consider taking a lot of fluids and water. Try and eat foods that are rich in fiber, as well as non-starchy vegetables. This helps to reduce constipation.

8. Changes in sleep

When you start your ketogenic lifestyle initially, you may notice some changes to your sleeping habits. Before you know it, you are waking up at night, or having problems sleeping. This is because your body is getting used to the new diet. Once all that change, you start to sleep well

9. Bad breath

One consequence of ketosis is ketosis breath. You may notice that you have metallic breath. This happens as a result of the ketones being ejected from your body through both your urine and breath. At times, you may see your breath metallic. Other times, it may be fruity.

You can brush your teeth multiple times in a day and use sugar-free gums. They can help. After a while, your breath returns to normal.

10. Better focus and concentration

Do you know that studies show that those who are subscribers to ketogenic lifestyle have better concentration and focus? Yes, you read that right.

At first, when you start the keto diet, you may notice headaches and tiredness. This is for short while as the body adapts to the diet. After a while, you no longer see the symptoms.

If you use a keto diet for a while and religiously follow, you will notice that your clarity level has improved. Before you know it, you become a lot of focus. A study on epileptic patient showed that those who took up the keto diet become alert and attentive. Before you know it, they didn't have to battle with alert issues.

It was noticed that their level of alertness in the cognitive tests they did improve.

Chapter Three

How Does It Work

A lot of persons use a ketogenic diet for one reason or the other. It could be to shed weight or to treat epilepsy or Alzheimer's disease. Whatever the case may be, you will face the same thing when you take a keto diet.

Immediately you cut down on your consumption of carbs; you tend to notice that the amount of carbs in your food has reduced.

Before you cut the carb, the body usually burnt glucose, a product of the carbs. When you take in the carb, it is digested into glucose and used as an energy source. The glucose is transported by the blood around the body, especially the brain and the cells. The brain uses up glucose as an energy source to function well. Since you are eating a lot of foods that are high in carbs, the body continues to store up fats. Before you know it, you are increasing in weight and size.

When you have had enough and decided to lose weight, you can try out the keto diet and combine it with exercise, though not compulsory. A lot of persons use both to force their bodies into a state of ketosis quickly and burn off the burnt fat.

When you embrace keto, you toss away those foods that are high in carbs and embrace those that are high in fats.

Whatever you do while on a keto diet, your foods should be high in fats, moderate in protein and low in carbs. Do not eat foods that are high in carbs because it could ruin your efforts. The body loves glucose, and immediately it sights high amount of carbs, even when it is in a state of ketosis, it throws the state of ketosis one side and embraces the glucose once more. When you eat foods that are high in protein, it is bad, as the body can transform excess protein to glucose.

What Happens When You Take Keto Friendly Diet

At first, when you consume a keto diet, you may notice keto flu. What is that? It is common to see a lot of those who are new to the ketogenic lifestyle feel some flu-like symptoms. Why does this happen?

When you take foods high in fats, and low in carbs, the body tries to adapt to the change. This means that the body won't have access to glucose any longer. The brain will try to adapt to its new energy source, ketones, and this can lead to headaches and nausea.

It could be as a result of you using the loo a lot. When a person is new to keto, he or she tends to urinate a lot. Why? It is simple. The person is losing a lot of electrolytes and water, hence needs replacement. You take a lot of water, as it can help.

Once you start reducing the number of carbs you take, the body, especially the liver takes the fats consumed and turn them to ketones and fatty acid. The ketones are the energy source, and they take the place of glucose. They are used by the body to carry out their daily activities. That's not all, as the body starts to use the stored up fats. You see all those stored up fats that once remained untouched; the body starts to convert them to ketones. Before you know it, you are shedding weight effortlessly. At this stage, you are in ketosis. To prevent yourself from falling out of this state, you need to keep eating what you are eating.

Chapter Four

Top 10 Foods You Need to Avoid

While you decide to embrace the ketogenic diet for one reason or the other, whether to shed weight or not, it is important to note that you should avoid some unhealthy foods. The one that tops the list are foods high in carbs. As much as we want you to eat foods that are high in carbs, we advise that you avoid those that have unhealthy fats like margarine. Whatever food high in fat that you cook must be healthy fats.

To prevent your body from falling out of the prided ketosis that took you weeks to get into, there are some foods that you should consider avoiding, and they are:

1. High-carb sauces

You see those sauces that you used while eating high carbs foods; they should be avoided. When you walk into the grocery store to buy a sauce, it is important to check it is keto friendly and without sugar. Some sauces that you should be cautious about are sweet salad dressing, barbecue sauce, as well as dipping sauces.

2. Bread and baked products

It is important to clamp down on the number of baked products that you consume. Many of them are high in carbs like a doughnut, rolls, white bread, cookies, crackers and so on. If you must eat baked products, ensure that they are made from keto friendly ingredients.

3. Pasta

When you jump onto the keto train, you will have to do away with noodles and spaghetti. Those foods are packing a lot of carbs. If you calculate the carbs that they have, you will be scared. If you are sure about losing weight, drop them.

4. Sweets.

There is hardly a soul on earth that doesn't fancy sweets. They are appealing to the taste buds and make us happy. We all know that, but they are high in carbs. While losing weight, they need to be tossed aside. Avoid things like maple syrup, candy, coconut sugar, and agave syrup. Your body will thank you to that.

5. Grain products

Try and toss the grain aside. A lot of these cereals that you consume in the morning are so high in carbs that if consumed can ruin your keto journey. You should think of tossing your oats, rice, and wheat aside. Kiss goodbye to tortillas and you will be happy for it.

6. Sweetened beverages.

Sweet! We love sweet things. We love our soda, sports drinks, sweetened teas, and juice. A lot of us can't do without them, but they are dangerous to health.

7. Starchy vegetables.

Veggies are good, but starchy veggies should be avoided while working on losing your weight. They trump whatever progress that you have made with your keto diet. You should think of tossing foods like pumpkin, peas, corn, and potatoes aside.

Eat veggies that are low in carbs and your weight loss will surprise you.

8. Beans and legumes.

You can increase the rate of your body burning fat by trying to avoid foods that are very high in protein. You want foods that are moderate in protein. Why? You may ask. When the body doesn't see carbs, and it sees a high amount of protein, it turns that amount to glucose.

Avoid foods like kidney beans, lentils, chickpeas, and black beans.

9. Alcoholic beverages.

Alcoholic beverages and keto do not go in the same sentence except when they negate each other. The truth remains that alcoholic beverages have a high amount of carbs. If you want to save yourself the stress, you should consider avoiding them.

10. Fruit.

While on your journey to losing weight, we advise that you take fruits, but we also advise that you avoid some fruits because of their carb level. Check the carb level of fruit before you take it. Some fruits to avoid are pineapple, bananas, grapes, and citrus.

Chapter Five

Errors to avoid

The journey to losing weight can be a simple one if you understand what to do and what time. It is common to see a lot of persons wallowing in one problem or the other because they made an error. Getting into a state of ketosis is not a day's journey, and when you leave that state because of an error on your part, getting into it becomes a problem. It is advisable to know these errors and try to avoid them. The results will surprise you.

Eating enough fat.

As much as you know the keto diet has low carb content, it is important to complement it with high fat content. About seventy percent of what you consume should be healthy fats, while five percent should be carbs, and the remaining twenty percent should be protein.

When you eat fat, you will realize that you will be satisfied. Hence your carb cravings reduce. This allows you to remain in the state of ketosis.

Eating too much protein.

A lot of persons feel that once they reduce carbs, and consume a high amount of fats that they can eat a lot of protein. This is one error that should be avoided.

When you eat an excess amount of protein, one thing is sure; it is transformed into glucose using the process of gluconeogenesis.

This means that you are indirectly eating carbs. As much as you should eat a low carb diet, the protein content should be low too. We are not excluding carbs from the diet; we are just restricting it to the amount that some body parts like blood cells need to survive. If you eat a lot of protein, you have merely given the body excess protein that it could turn to glucose.

Eating hidden carbs without realizing it.

One thing that should be noted is that some foods have carbs that you do not know of. It is common to see some condiments possessing hidden carbs.

Before you buy any food, look at its label, and try to see if there is any hidden sugar. It won't take a long time to check. This can determine if you succeed or fail in your keto journey.

Not sleeping enough.

Once you have decided to get enough sleep, you are getting closer to shedding weight. Do you know that a lot of persons feel that starving themselves of sleep improve their chances of shedding weight? This is a pure fallacy. When you don't sleep, your body becomes stressed, which reduces the level of metabolism.

Before you know it, you are storing up a lot of fats. When you are fatigued because you didn't sleep, you will notice that you will want to take latte to get a boost of energy. You may also want to dine in a late snack.

It is advisable to try and get about eight hours of sleep every night, as it helps to burn fats.

Eating too many keto sweets.

A lot of persons feel that eating a lot of keto brownies, and cookies are great because they are keto friendly, and have low carbs. You see them stuffing themselves with a lot of them. Can we burst your bubbles? The fact that they have low carbs doesn't mean that you should eat a lot of them. When you eat a lot of keto sweets with low carbs, you end up eating a lot of calories. That's not all, as you created for those sweet things before you know it, you are munching on sweets high in carbs.

You should eat keto sweets once in a while.

Snacking too much.

There are currently awesome snacks that you can eat while on a ketogenic diet like nuts, avocado, and cheese. This doesn't mean that you should eat them every time because at the end, you may add a lot of calories to your body, and you will realize that you aren't losing weight.

You should eat snacks only when you notice that you are very hungry in between meals. Apart from that, stay away from them.

Not replenishing your electrolytes.

When some persons begin the keto diet, they start to feel sick, having flu symptoms. The reasons this occurs are:

When the body is no longer using glucose as its energy source, and now has to use fat, the brain has to adapt to it. This may lead to headaches and nausea.

You may be dehydrated because you will urinate a lot while on keto. If you don't drink water, this can bring a lot of issues.

If you notice the keto flu, don't be scared. This shows that your body is adapting to the keto diet. What you should do to reduce the keto flu is to take a lot of water. You need to have your electrolytes supplemented

One supplement that you should consider taking to put you in the right state is KetoLogic

BHB. It helps to treat the keto flu and ushers you quickly into ketosis.

Eating too much dairy.

A lot of persons tend to have an inflammatory response when they consume a lot of dairy products. This can affect their progress to weight loss. That's not all, like we earlier said, taking a lot of protein can inhibit weight loss.

A lot of dairy foods have both protein and fats. Some even have carbs but in a limited amount.

When you consume dairy foods, ensure that its fat content is higher than its protein and carbs content.

Eating too many calories.

A lot of persons think that one can consume as much as they want, as long as the food is keto friendly. This is misleading and should be avoided at all costs.

You should consume healthy fats in large quantity, but you should never eat more calories that can be burnt. If you eat excess food, the additional calories end up as body fat.

Usually, a normal person needs close to two thousand calories daily, but this number is dependent on some factors like activity, height, and gender.

Not drinking enough water.

Our basic health science class taught us that water is key to our health. If you fall under those that hate taking water, then there is a big problem because your rate of metabolism will drop.

You should try and take about sixty-four ounces of water daily. This helps to remove the toxins. While you start your keto journey, you need to drink a lot of water, as it helps to combat the keto flu and so on.

Chapter Six

The best ten foods you need

While on keto, some foods should be eaten, and there are some that should be avoided. Below are ten foods that you should consider eating while on a keto diet:

Nuts and Seeds

Have you tried the sunflower seeds, pumpkin seeds, macadamia nuts, almonds, and pecans? They are all awesome ways that one can get healthy fats.

They are high in fiber and without a high amount of carbs. They are easy to afford, and you can easily track your carbs with them.

You can use them as snacks or even add them to the ingredients of smoothies.

Olives

Have you tried black and green olives? They are high in healthy fats, and great for the heart. Since you are in keto, you need foods that are high in fats and low in carbs. Olives can offer you this. You can easily have them warmed up with the marinara, or even garnish zoodles with it.

Condiments

A lot of things that you will find in the condiments aisles are keto friendly, though you have to read their labels first to be sure. Some options that you consider looking at are:

- Mayo

- Ketchup

- Buffalo sauce

- Salad dressing

- Mustard.

Oils

Whatever oil you decide to buy, it is important to check if they are made up of fat. As much as keto preaches eating foods that are high in fats, they also want you to consume those that are high in healthy fats.

Some of the oils that you can consider using are:

- Coconut oil

- MCT oil

- Cooking oil- Don't forget to look at the label.

- Noncooking oil- Don't forget to look at the label.

Ghee

Yes, you read that right! Clarified butter or ghee is great for keto. You can use the shrimp, asparagus, and butter to give that saltiness that you wish for.

A lot of persons are in love with ghee, as it gives off the nuttiness unseen in usual butter. It is great to the taste buds.

Salt

You need salt. Everyone that undergoes ketogenic lifestyle needs salt. Why is this so? When your body starts to burn fat, you may tend to feel the electrolyte swings.

Before you know it, you can't stop urinating constantly. What this means is that your body is shedding a lot of electrolytes and sodium.

Taking salt helps to replace it.

Prepared Snacks

Who said you couldn't have snacks while on Keto? No one. What you can't have are processed or unhealthy snacks. Do you feel like snacking? You can munch on snacks that aren't high in carbs like

- Cheese crisps
- Pork rinds
- Pill nuts
- Meat snacks.

Flours and Thickeners

You can use keto friendly flour to bake. You don't have to stop baking just because you are on a keto diet. You can try the almond meal, almond flour, as well as coconut flour. They have a low carb, but high in fiber.

Since they come with a nutty flavor, they are great for waffles, muffins, pancakes or even cookies.

Nut Butter

A lot of traditional peanut butter comes with sugar. There is the unsweetened option that can be consumed by keto eaters. You will enjoy peanut butter without pumping yourself with lots of sugar.

You can also have access to the unsweetened almond butter. You can also make your own. Add vanilla or cinnamon to it, and you will enjoy it

Keto-approved Sweeteners

When people think of healthy living, they think of bland foods. Gone are those days when you had to eat tasteless things all in the name of following the keto lifestyle. If you love the thought of consuming pancakes, you can try it out with keto friendly sweeteners like Swerve, Splenda, Stevia and so on.

Chapter Seven

Keto-friendly recipes

Chorizo breakfast bake

What You Need

- Olive oil- A tbsp

- Red pepper- Half cup

- Onion- Half cup

- Chorizo sausages- Four oz

- Eggs- Two

- Pepper

- Salt

- Bacon- Two slices

Guidelines

Start by preheating the oven to a high temperature of 250. Try and grease the two ramekins.

Take out a skillet and place it on a stove with medium heat.

Whisk in your onion and peppers. Allow them to cook for about five minutes till you notice that they have been browned.

Have the veggies mixture shared among the two ramekins.

Have the chorizo chopped, then shared them between the ramekins.

Break the egg, and put it in every ramekin. Add the pepper, as well as the salt.

Have it baked for about twelve minutes till you notice that the egg is ready.

Have the bacon crumbled on the top. You can only serve it hot.

Cheesy single-serve Lasagna

What You Need

- Marinara- Three tbsp
- Zucchini- One
- Ricotta cheese- Two tbsp
- Mozzarella- Three oz

Guidelines

Take out a bowl that is microwave safe, then add a spoonful of the marinara sauce.

Take out the sauce and spread it on the zucchini slices. Use a tbsp of the ricotta on it.

Do the same with the other layers, as well as ricotta and sauce.

Use the other zucchini to cover it, then add the mozzarella.

Leave in the microwave for about four minutes till they are well heated, and the cheese has melted.

Mushroom Soup with Fried egg

What You Need

- Olive oil- One Tsp

- Mushrooms- Four

- Cauliflower- One hundred grams

- Vegetable broth- One cup

- Heavy cream- Three tbsp

- Cheese- Two tbsp

- Butter- One Tsp

- Egg- One

Guidelines

Take out your saucepan, and put it on a stove with medium heat. Have the oil heated.

Toss in the mushrooms, then allow them to cook till you notice they are soft. This should take six minutes.

Add your heavy cream, veggie broth, as well as riced cauliflower.

Toss in the pepper and salt. Whisk in your cheese.

Allow the soup simmer, till it has thickened to the extent that it is necessary. Then take it off the state be.

Try and have the egg fried in the butter to the extent that you want. It can be served with the soup.

Avocado Egg & salami sandwiches

What You Need

- Cloud buns- Four

- Eggs- Four

- Butter- One Tsp

- Tomato- One

- Mozzarella- One oz

- Avocado- One

- Pepper

- Salt

- Two oz of sliced salami

Guidelines

Take out the baking sheet, and line it.

Have the cloud buns put there, then leave it in an oven. Allow it there till they become golden brown.

Take out a big skillet, and put it on a stove with medium heat, then add the butter there.

Break the eggs and put them in the skillet, before you try to season them with pepper, as well as salt.

Allow the eggs to cook to the extent that they are ready, then put on every cloud bun.

Add the tomato slice, avocado, mozzarella, as well as salami on the buns.

Serve now.

Mozzarella Tuna Melt

What You Need

- Olive oil- One tbsp

- Onion- Half cup

- Mayo- Quarter cup

- Tuna- Eight oz

- Eggs- Two

- Mozzarella- Two oz

- Pepper

- Salt

- Onion- One

Guidelines

Have the skillet placed on a stove with medium heat. Put the oil there, then whisk in the onion. Allow it to cook for close to five minutes.

Have the tuna drained, then allow it flaked in the skillet. Continue to whisk in the rest of the ingredients.

Add your pepper and salt. Whisk them, and allow them to cook for about two minutes. The cheese should have melted.

Take out a bowl, and add the green onion. You can serve.

Three-cheese Pizza Frittata

What You Need

- Thawed Frozen Spinach- Ten oz

- Eggs- Six

- Olive oil- Two tbsp

- Italian seasoning- Half tsp

- Pepper

- Salt

- Ricotta cheese- Quarter cup

- Parmesan cheese- Quarter cup

- Mozzarella cheese- Two and a half oz

- Pepperoni- One oz

Guidelines

Have the oven preheated to a high temperature of 175. Take out the pie plate, then grease using cooking spray.

Have the spinach defrosted. Do this by leaving it in a microwave for about four minutes. This will drive out the water.

Break the egg, then add the olive oil, pepper, salt, and Italian seasoning. Whisk them well.

Add the parmesan cheese, ricotta cheese, as well as drained spinach, then whisk them till they form well.

Toss in a pie plate, the mixture that was formed. Add the pepperoni, as well as mozzarella.

Leave in the oven for about forty minutes. By this time, the egg has been set, while the cheese has been browned a bit.

You can then serve.

Bacon Breakfast Bombs

What You Need

- Bacon- Four slices

- Eggs- Two

- Butter- Quarter cup

- Mayo- Two tbsp

- Pepper

- Salt

Guidelines

Take out a large skillet and place it on a stove with medium heat. Put the bacon there till they become crisp.

Allow the bacon to rest for a while before you chop it. Keep the bacon grease somewhere else.

Take out a saucepan, and put water in it, then add salt. Allow it boil well.

Put the eggs there, then allow them to boil for about ten minutes. Place them in a water bath.

Allow the eggs to rest. You can then peel them well. Don't forget to cut them coarsely.

Have the eggs mashed, then whisk the butter, pepper, salt, and mayo.

Whisk the bacon grease that was kept somewhere, before you have the mixture covered. Allow them to chill for half an hour.

Have the egg mixture shared into the portion before you have them rolled into the balls. Don't forget to have them rolled in the crushed bacon.

Try and serve it instantly. The ones that are leftovers, store in the refrigerator.

Easy Cloud Buns

What You Need

- Eggs- Three

- Cream of tartar- One-eight tsp

- Cream cheese- Three oz.

Guidelines

Have the oven preheated to a high temperature of 200. Take out your baking sheet and line it up using parchment.

Whisk your egg whites till you notice that they are foamy, then you can add the cream of tartar. Whisk them well till you see that the egg whites are both opaque and shiny, showing soft peaks.

Take out a different bowl, and add the egg yolks and cream cheese. Whisk them well, and then add the egg white mixture.

On your baking sheet, put the batter and make quarter cup circles. Leave close to two inches between both of them.

Allow them to bake for about half an hour, till you notice that the buns are no longer soft.

You can then serve.

Gyro Salad With Avo-tzatziki

Prep Time: 10 minutes

What You Need

- Olive oil- A tbsp
- Lamb meat- One pound
- Onion- Half
- Chicken broth- Quarter cup

- Lemon juice- Four tsp

- Dried oregano- Half tsp

- Dried thyme- Half tsp

- Cucumber- Half

- Avocado- One

- Mint- Half tsp

- Dill- One Tsp

- Romaine lettuces- Six cups

Guidelines

Take out your big skillet, then put it on a stove with medium heat. Put the oil there, then the lamb.

Allow them to cook for about three minutes, and toss well. You can add your onion now.

Continue to cook well till the lamb is well cooked. Add the onion there, then whisk them well, before you add the thyme, oregano, lemon juice, and chicken broth.

Add the pepper, as well as the salt. Allow it simmer well for about five minutes.

Have the cucumber grated well, before you use a clean towel to remove the moisture of any kind.

Put the cucumber into the food processor, before you toss in the lemon juice, salt, dill, mint, as well as avocado. Continue until they become smooth.

Have them served.

Cabbage and Sausage Skillet

What You Need

- Sausage links- Six

- Cabbage- Half

- Butter- Two tbsp

- Sour cream- Quarter cup

- Mayo- Quarter cup

- Pepper

- Salt

Guidelines

Take out a skillet, and place it on a stove with medium heat. Put the sausage there till they are browned well. Remove the sausage, and slice well.

Put the skillet in the stove on medium heat again, then toss the butter into it.

Add your cabbage, then whisk till it becomes wilted. This should take over four minutes.

Whisk in the sausage that has been stirred in the wilted cabbage. Add your mayo, as well as sour cream.

Toss the pepper, as well as salt. Allow them to simmer for about ten minutes.

You can serve well.

Chicken Zoodle Alfredo

What You Need

- Chicken breasts- Six oz

- Olive oil- One tbsp

- Pepper

- Salt

- Butter- Two tbsp

- Heavy cream- Quarter cup

- Parmesan cheese- Quarter cup

- Zucchini- Two hundred grams.

Guidelines

Have the skillet placed on a stove with medium

heat. Put the oil there.

Add the pepper, as well as salt to the chicken. Toss the chicken to the heated skillet.

Have them cooked for about six minutes till it is cooked. Have the chicken cut into strips.

Put the skillet on the stove on the medium heat again, then toss the butter.

Add your parmesan cheese, as well as heavy cream. Allow them to become thick.

Have the zucchini spiralized before you toss it in the mixture that has the chicken.

Continue to cook the zucchini until it becomes soft. It should take over three minutes. Try and serve it hot.

Pan-fried Pepperoni Pizzas

What You Need

- Eggs- Six

- Parmesan cheese- Six tbsp

- Psyllium husk powder- Three tbsp

- Italian seasoning- One and a half tsp

- Olive oil- Three tbsp

- Tomato sauce- Nine tbsp

- Mozzarella- Four and a half oz

- Pepperoni- One and a half oz

- Chopped basil- Three tbsp

Guidelines

Take out a blender, and toss in the parmesan, eggs, Italian seasoning, psyllium husk powder, as well as salt.

Continue to blend well till you notice that it smooth. This should take close to a minute. Allow it to rest well for about five minutes.

Take out a skillet and place it on a stove with medium heat. Add a tbsp of oil.

Have one-third of the batter added to the skillet. Allow them to spread into a circle, and then brown well.

Have the pizza crust flipped, till it becomes brown.

Take off the crust and put it in the baking sheet. Do it over and over again using the extra batter.

Add three tbsp of the tomato sauce on every crust.

Add the cheese and pepperoni. Allow them to broil till you notice that the cheese has been browned.

Add your basil. Slice before you serve.

Easy Cheeseburger Salad

What You Need

- Beef- Seven oz

- Mayo- Three tbsp

- Pepper

- Salt

- Pickles- One tbsp

- Mustard- One Tsp

- Ketchup- Half tsp

- Smoked paprika

- Romaine lettuce- Three oz

- Tomatoes- One-third cup

- Cheddar cheese- Quarter cup

Guidelines

Have the ground beef browned. You can then add the pepper and salt.

Try and remove the fat from the beef. Take it out of the heat.

Take out a blender, and add the paprika, ketchup, mustard, pickles, and mayo.

Have the mixture blended well.

Take out a bowl, and add the cheddar cheese, tomatoes, lettuce, and ground beef.

Coat dressing gently on it. You can then serve.

Pepper Jack Sausage Egg Muffins

What You Need

- Ground sausage- Ten oz
- Garlic powder- Quarter tsp
- Onion- Half cup
- Pepper
- Salt
- Eggs- Three
- Heavy cream- Two tbsp
- Pepper Jack Cheese- Half cup

Guidelines

Have the oven preheated to a high temperature of 250. Take out the three ramekins and grease them well using cooking spray.

Take out a bowl, and add the pepper, salt, garlic powder, onion, and ground sausage.

Have the sausage mix shared well using the ramekins. Have them pressed into the sides, as well as the bottom. Allow the middle to be opened.

Have the eggs whisked, then toss the pepper, salt, and heavy cream.

Have the egg mixture shared in the sausage cups, then toss the shredded chess.

Leave them in the oven for about thirty minutes till the eggs have been set. Ensure that the cheese is browned.

You can then serve.

Mozzarella Veggie-loaded Quiche

What You Need

- Almond flour- Six tbsp

- Parmesan cheese- One tbsp

- Eggs- Two

- Bacon- Two

- Frozen spinach- Quarter cup

- Zucchini- Quarter cup

- Mozzarella cheese- Quarter cup

- Tomatoes- Four

- Heavy cream- One tbsp

- Chives- One Tsp

Guidelines

Take out a bowl, and whisk in the parmesan and almond flour. Toss in the salt and egg. Whisk well till it becomes soft.

Take out a quiche pan, and ensure that the dough is pressed. Allow it to be spread evenly.

Have the sides, as well as bottom scored. Allow the dough bake for about seven minutes. It should be heated to a high temperature of 225.

Take it out and allow it cool well.

Take out a skillet, and brown the bacon with it, then place it in a quiche pan.

Have zucchini, spinach, tomatoes, and cheese sprinkled there.

Have the remaining egg whisked with chives, heavy cream, salt, and pepper. Add the mixture poured in the quiche.

Allow it to bake for about twenty-five minutes till the egg has been set.

Savory Ham And Cheese Waffles

What You Need

- Eggs- Four

- Egg White Protein Powder- Two scoops

- Baking powder- One Tsp

- Butter- One-third cup

- Salt- half tsp

- Ham- One oz

- Cheddar cheese- Quarter cup

Guidelines

Break two eggs, and beat their yolks, then add the baking powder, protein, salt, and butter using a bowl.

Add the cheddar cheese and chopped ham to the mixture.

Take out another bowl, and beat in the egg whites, as well as the salt till you notice the stiff peaks forming.

Toss in the egg whites that have been beaten to the egg yolk mixture in two different batches.

Take out your waffle maker, and preheat it before you grease it. Add a quarter batter cup before you close it.

Continue to cook till you notice that the waffle has turned a golden brown hue. This should take close to four minutes. You can remove them.

Have the waffle maker reheated, then do the same with the other batter.

Have the oil in that skillet heated; have your eggs fried with pepper and salt.

You can then serve the hot waffles. Don't forget to top it using fried egg.

Chapter Eight

Tips for losing 21 pounds in 21 days

Losing those pounds do not have to be stressful as long as you know what you are doing. With these tips, you get closer to shedding twenty-one pounds in twenty-one days. The great aspect of them is that they can easily be done.

Drink A Lot Of Water

This is something that shouldn't be ignored. You have to gulp down as much water as possible. It is really bad that a lot of persons hate drinking water. The major source of liquid to them is alcohol or soft drinks. Taking a lot of water helps the body to remove those toxins, improve on digestion, clamp down on constipation and to bloat. It even goes ahead to improve metabolism and internal PH. It is advisable to drink about four liters of water daily.

When you wake up in the morning, one of the first things you should do apart from brushing your teeth is to drink at least two glasses of water that's at room temperature. It is advisable to add fenugreek seeds to it, as they help to improve the metabolism.

You can try to create homemade detox water by tossing in mint leaves, cumin, garlic, and cucumber. This allows the body to function well.

Stop Eating Junk Food, Sugar And Processed Food

This is definitely for your good. Try and avoid junk foods of all kind for three weeks. When watching Netflix at night, don't be tempted to munch on the sugar. Don't worry, do it for three weeks without cheating, and you will be amazed by the awesome results you will notice.

Throw away every type of unhealthy food that is laced with sugar, preservatives and a large amount of sodium. What should be in your kitchen are low calories foods and whole foods.

If the craving for sugary things come, opt for yogurts that are low in calories, and top them with peaches or figs.

Try and add a piece of dark chocolate once you are done with dinner. It can help with the craving.

Eat Different Kinds of Fruits and Veggies

On your journey to shedding pounds, it is advisable to try out different kinds of veggies and fruits. I will advise you to try out three kinds of fruits, and five kinds of vegetables daily. Why is this so? When you consume veggies and fruits, you introduce a high amount of minerals, vitamins, dietary fiber, as well as phytonutrients to the body. They go a long way to improve the level of satiety while reducing the rate of absorption of those fat molecules.

Veggies and fruits have little calories and can enhance the movement of your bowel, while your body builds its immunity level. As your body cells improve in their functioning, your stored up fat is used as an energy source. Before you know it, you are losing weight.

Avoid White Carbs

When we talk of bad carbs or white carbs, we are speaking of delicacies such as sugar, flour, crackers, white rice, cereals, and pasta. When you look at these foods, one thing is sure- they are highly refined and come bearing little nutrients. Their calorie level shoots through the roof. When you munch on bad carbs, the level of your glucose level increase. Since they are digested quickly, before you know it, you are hungry again and munching on those high-calorie meals.

You should try out healthier varieties such as beans, cauliflower, turnip, and white potatoes.

Eat On Time and Reduce the amount of food you munch on

When I hear people complain that they don't eat early or starve for a long time, yet their weight seems to be increasing, I know that those methods are futile. Starving and not eating on time shouldn't be what you use when you want to shed weight.

What you should do is to eat on time and control the size of the food you consume. Do you know that the amount of food you eat adds a lot too if you gain weight or not.

One thing that you should know is that you may have a healthy eating habit, but if your body is unable to digest, absorb, as well as remove toxins quickly, your entire system may have a huge problem to deal with.

This could worsen into a slow metabolism, thereby improving the blood glucose, as well as blood pressure. Before you know it, your weight is increasing.

This is why you should try and eat breakfast, and dinner before night. Don't try eating snacks late, and ensure you rest well.

When you starve yourself, your body enters famine mode, thereby forcing the body cells to keep everything eaten into a state of fat. When the hunger comes at night, you can munch on fruits instead of snacks. Like always, don't forget to drink lots of water.

Watch How You Eat

I mean you should do it. You are probably wondering why we asked you to do this. Well, take a ride with us. It is important to note that these tips are short term ones to make you lose the necessary weight.

When you sit in front of a mirror and watch yourself eat, you stop overeating. While you eat, try and shut your mouth as you chew. This prevents you from taking in air and improves the functioning of your digestive system.

While you serve yourself, opt for a smaller plate and spoon, as they prevent you from eating a lot of food. Try and eat gradually, and eliminate all forms of distractions such as watching TV, using the phone and so on.

Work It Out

One thing that you should note is that when you lose weight quickly, you may gain the weight back, and come bearing loose skin.

To look healthy and toned, if it is advisable that you start exercising. If you don't fancy running or the gym, you should think of trying yoga. You can as well swim or even dance.

If you love the gym, you can consider trying bodyweight training, and maybe, you can flaunt that cute body you worked on at the beach.

When you work out, your metabolism increases, and you will be able to sleep well. If you want to work on your confidence, you should consider working on.

Get Your Beauty Sleep

A lot of persons feel that when they sleep a lot, they will gain weight. That's a pure fallacy, as the opposite is the case. Not sleeping well can improve your weight gain. If you don't sleep for about eight hours, your body cells won't be able to process the food properly. They won't be able to get rid of those toxins. When you rarely sleep, your healing process reduces, and you become a lot stressed.

Before you know it, you are gaining a lot of weight, and fatigued, even when you have not carried out anything throughout the day.

Chapter Nine

21-day meal plan shopping list

Are you thinking of starting a ketogenic diet, and wondering what to eat? This 21-day meal plan can help.

Day 1

For breakfast, try out the Chorizo Breakfast Bake.

For lunch, you can try out the Sesame Pork Lettuce Wraps.

For dinner, you can try out the Avocado Lime Salmon.

The total calories of the food for day 1 are 1,520. As for fat, it is 109g.

For protein, it is 110g. The net carbs of the foods are 16g.

Day 2

For breakfast, consume the leftover chorizo breakfast bake.

For lunch, try out the Thick Cut Bacon with spiced pumpkin soup leftover

For dinner, try out the Avocado Lime Salmon.

The total calories of the foods are 1,570. As for fat, it is 124g. For protein, it is 92g, and the net carbs are 16g.

Day 3

For breakfast, try out Baked Eggs in Avocado.

For lunch, try out Easy Beef Curry Rosemary.

For dinner, try out Roasted Chicken and Veggies.

The total calories are 1,700. As for fat, it is 128.5g. As for protein, it is 103g, and the net carbs are 22g.

Day 4

For breakfast, try out the Lemon Poppy Ricotta, pancakes and three slices of bacon.

For lunch, try out the pumpkin soup, avocado.

For dinner, try out the roasted chicken and veggies that were left over.

The total calories of the day's foods are 1,665. As for fat, it is 130g. For protein, it is 95.5g, and the net carbs for the day are 23.5g.

Day 5

For breakfast, try out the lemon poppy ricotta pancakes, as well as the thick cut bacon.

For lunch, try out the porridge and bacon.

For dinner, try out the leftover beef curry, as well as cheesy sausage and mushroom skillet.

The total calories of the foods are 1,670. For fat, it is 112g, protein is 100g, and net carbs are 33.5g.

Day 6

For breakfast, try out the sweet blueberry coconut porridge that was left over.

For lunch, try out the Easy beef curry.

For dinner, try out the lamb chops and garlic, and Rosemary.

The total calories of the foods are 1,625. For fat, it is 108g; protein is 110.5g.

Shopping List For The First Week

For the Protein, you should consider shopping for the following:

Seventeen slices of bacon

A pound of the beef

Four chicken thighs, deskinned and boneless.

Four oz of Chorizo sausages

Seven eggs

Two lamb chops

Six oz pork

Six oz Italian sausage

DAIRY

A cup of almond milk

A pound of butter

Two tbsps of cheddar cheese

Five tbsps of heavy creams

Half cup of mozzarella cheese

Six oz of ricotta cheese

PRODUCE

A quarter pound of asparagus

Two avocados

Small green bell pepper

Medium red bell pepper

Sixty grams of blueberries

Four leaves of butter lettuce

Two carrots

One stalk of celery

A bunch of cilantro

One head of garlic

One piece of ginger

One lemon

One lime

Four oz mushrooms

Two onion

One parsnip

One rosemary

One zucchini

FOR PANTRY ITEMS

- A quarter cup of almond flour
- Balsamic vinegar
- Baking powder
- One cup of chicken broth

- A quarter cup of coconut flour

- One coconut milk can

- Curry powder

- Coconut oil

- Dried thyme

- Dried oregano

- Garlic powder

- Egg white protein powder

- Liquid Stevia

- Olive oil

- A quarter cup of marinara sauce

- Pepper

- Onion powder

- Half cup of Pumpkin puree

- One tbsp of Poppy seeds

- Salt

- Powdered erythritol

- One tbsp of sesame seeds

- Sesame oil

- A quarter cup of shaved coconut

Day 7

For breakfast, try out the far busting vanilla protein smoothy

For lunch, try out the cheeseburger salad.

For dinner, try out the chicken zoodle Alfredo. The total calories of the foods are 1,530. For fat, it is 113.5g, protein is 107.5g, and the net carbs are 18.5g.

Day 8

For breakfast, try out the ham and cheese.

For lunch, try out the waffles and bacon.

For dinner, try out the pepperoni pizzas cabbage, as well as sausage skillet.

The total calories of the foods are 1,670.

For fat, it is 129g, protein is 103g, and the net carbs are 20.5g.

Day 9

For breakfast, try out the three cloud buns and three tablespoons of peanut butter, as well as bacon.

For lunch, try out the Three-Cheese Pizza Frittata and bacon.

For dinner, try out the pepperoni, ham, as well as bacon.

For lunch, try out the Three-Cheese Pizza Frittata and bacon.

For dinner, try out the pepperoni, ham, as well as Cheddar Stromboli.

The total calories of the foods are 1,640.

For fat, it is 130.5g, protein is 100.5g, and the net carbs are 20.5g.

Day 10

For breakfast, try out the mozzarella veggie loaded.

For lunch, try out the quiche, bacon, cheeseburger salad.

For dinner, try out the gyro salad and

Avo-tzatziki. The total calories of the foods are 1,580. For fat, it is 104.5g, protein is 117.5g, and the net carbs are 33g.

Day 11

For breakfast, try out the Pepper Jack Sausage, egg muffins and bacon.

For lunch, try out the pepperoni pizza.

For dinner, try out the cabbage and sausage skillet that was left over.

The total calories are 1,650. For fat, it is 127.5g, protein is 101g, and the net carbs are 29g.

Day 12

For breakfast, try out the ham and cheese waffles, and bacon.

For lunch, try out the cabbage and sausage skillet.

For dinner, try out the chicken zoodle Alfredo. The total calories of the foods are 1,620. For fat, it is 119g, protein is 119g, and the net carbs are 18.5g.

Day 13

For breakfast, try out pepper jack sausage egg muffins and bacon.

For lunch, try out the pepperoni pizza that is left over.

For dinner, try out the gyro salad and Avo-Tzatziki that are left over.

The total calories of the foods are 1,595. For fat, it is 116g, protein is 110g, and the net carbs are 15.5g.

Day 14

For breakfast, try out the pepper jack sausage egg muffins and half avocado.

For lunch, try out the cabbage, sausage skills, and bacon.

For dinner, try out the gyro salad and Avo-Tzatziki.

The total calories of the foods are 1,605. For fat, it is 102g, protein is 102g, and net carbs are 22.5g.

Shopping List

PROTEIN

You need the following to make your second-week meals:

- Eleven Bacon

- Seven oz beef

- Ten ounces sausage

- Six oz chicken breast

- Fifteen eggs

- One oz ham

- One pound lamb

- One and a half oz pepperoni

- Six sausage links

DAIRY

- For dairy, try the following:

- A quarter cup of almond milk

- A three-quarter cup of butter

- Half cup of cheddar cheese

- One cup of heavy cream

- Half cup of mayo

- One and a half cups of mozzarella cheese

- Three-quarter of parmesan cheese

- Half cup of pepper jack cheese

- A quarter cup of sour cream

- A quarter cup of whipped cream

PRODUCE

- Two avocados

- One Basil

- Half head of cabbage

- One chive

- One cucumber

- One dill

- One lemon

- One mint

- One onion

- Seven and half cups of romaine lettuce

- Quarter cup of frozen spinach

- Four tomatoes

- One-third of tomatoes

- Two cups of zucchini

PANTRY ITEMS

- Six tbsp of almond flour

- Quarter cup of chicken broth

- Baking powder

- Dried thyme

- Dried oregano

- Coconut oil

- Three scoops of vanilla

- Egg white protein powder,

- Italian season

- Garlic powder

- Olive oil

- Mustard

- Ketchup

- Black pepper

- Smoked paprika

- Salt

- Erythritol

- Psyllium husk powder

- Low car tomato sauce, and

- Vanilla extract

Day 15

For breakfast, try out the three tablespoons of peanut butter, three cloud buns, as well as bacon.

For lunch, try out the mozzarella tuna.

For dinner, try out the cheesy single serve lasagna.

The total calories are 1,605. For fat, it is 116.5g. For protein, it is 114.5g, and their net carbs are 28.5g.

Day 16

For breakfast, try out the Bacon Breakfast Bombs Avocado.

For lunch, try out the Egg & Salami Sandwiches.

For dinner, try out the Crispy Chipotle Chicken Thighs.

The total calories are 1,525. For fat, it is 118.5g, protein is 99.5g, and the net carbs are 12g.

Day 17

For breakfast, try out the Three-Cheese Pizza Frittata and Bacon.

For lunch, try out the mozzarella tuna melt.

For dinner, try out the Pepperoni, Ham, as well as Cheddar Stromboli.

The total calories are 1,660. For fat, it is 121g, protein is 119g, and net carbs are 22.5g.

Day 18

For breakfast, try out the three cloud buns and three tablespoons of peanut butter, as well as bacon.

For lunch, try out the Three-Cheese

Pizza Frittata and bacon.

For dinner, try out the pepperoni, ham, as well as bacon.

For lunch, try out the Three-Cheese

Pizza Frittata and bacon.

For dinner, try out the pepperoni, ham, as well as Cheddar Stromboli.

The total calories of the foods are 1,640.

For fat, it is 130.5g, protein is 100.5g, and the net carbs are 20.5g.

Day 19

For breakfast, try out the bacon breakfast bombs.

For lunch, try out the Avocado, Egg & Salami Sandwiches, as well as bacon.

For dinner, try out the Crispy Chipotle Chicken Thighs.

The total calories are 1,625. For fat, it is 126.5g, protein is 106.5g, and the net carbs are 12.5g.

Day 20

For breakfast, try out the Three-Cheese Pizza Frittata, and bacon.

For lunch, try out the Pepperoni, Ham, and Cheddar Stromboli.

For dinner, try out the Spring Salad with Steak and Sweet Dressing.

The total calories are 1,585.

For fat, it is 120.5g, protein is 108g, and the net carbs are 13.5g.

Day 21

For breakfast, try out the Three-Cheese Pizza Frittata and Bacon.

For lunch, try out the Mushroom Soup, as well as Fried Egg and bacon.

For dinner, try out the Spring Salad, Steak and Sweet Dressing are leftover.

The total calories are 1,665. For fat, it is 130.5g, protein is 110g, and the net carbs are 13.5g.

Shopping List

PROTEIN

- Twenty three bacon
- Seven oz of beef
- Twelve oz of chicken thighs
- Nineteen eggs
- Six oz of ham

- Three oz of pepperoni

- Two oz of salami

- Eight oz of tuna

DAIRY

- Seven tbsps of butter

- Two tbsps of shredded cheddar cheese

- Four oz of sliced cheddar cheese

- Three oz of cream cheese

- Three tbsp of heavy cream

- Six tbsp of mayo

- One oz of mozzarella

- Three and quarter mozzarella

- A quarter cup of parmesan cheese

- One-third of ricotta cheese.

PRODUCE

- One avocado

- One hundred grams of cauliflower

- One garlic

- Four mushrooms

- One green onion

- One onion

- Four raspberries

- Ten cups of salad greens

- Three cups of fresh spinach

- One frozen spinach

- One tomato

- One zucchini

PANTRY ITEMS

- A quarter cup of almond flour

- Chipotle Chili

- Baking powder

- Three tbsp of coconut flour

- Italian season

- Cream of tartar

- Almond flour

- Three tbsp marinara

- Liquid Stevia

- Ground coriander

- Garlic powder

- Onion powder

- Olive oil

- One oz of pine nuts

- Black pepper

- Salt

- Erythritol

- Paprika- Smoked

- One cup of vegetable broth, and

- White wine vinegar.

The recipes are in chapter 7.

Conclusion

When we are trying to lose weight, we become desperate to the extent that we are ready to swallow a lot of things. It is common to see some persons pumping themselves with pills, and at the end, they are left with one health issue or the other. What of those that try one product or the other that claims to work magic, and the end, money is gone, and the state has worsened. Are you tired of being duped? It is time you embraced the natural process and watch what you eat. The ketogenic diet can help you lose weight without you exercising, but if you want to speed it up, you can exercise.

Ingredients for keto foods are easy to stress, and the recipes are easy to make. You don't have to stress yourself any longer, all in the name of losing weight. The awesome part of all these is that keto friendly diets are tasteful to the taste buds. You don't have to sacrifice your love for sweet things on the altar of eating healthily.